Cookbook for beginner

Diabetic Diet

Delicious And Easy Recipes To Manage Your Diabetes Diet And Living Better With Diabetes

Gena miller

DIABETES

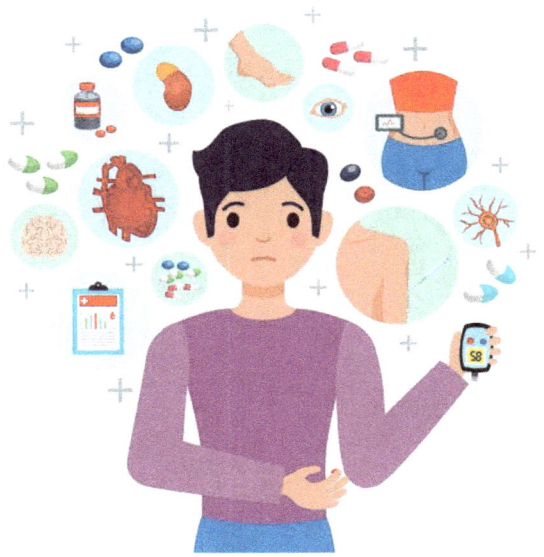

© Copyright 2021 by Gena Miller All rights reserved. The following Book is reproduced below with the goal of providing information that is as accurate and reliable as possible. Regardless, purchasing this Book can be seen as consent to the fact that both the publisher and the author of this book are in no way experts on the topics discussed within and that any recommendations or suggestions that are made herein are for entertainment purposes only. Professionals should be consulted as needed prior to undertaking any of the action endorsed herein. This declaration is deemed fair and valiby both the American Bar Association and the Committee of Publishers Association and is legally binding throughout the United States. Furthermore, the transmission, duplication, or reproduction of any of the following work including specific information will be considered an illegal act irrespective of if it is done electronically or in print. This extends to creating a secondary or tertiary copy of the work or a recorded copy and is only allowed with the express written consent from the Publisher. All additional right reserved. The information in the following pages is broadly considered a truthful and accurate account of facts and as such, any inattention, use, or misuse of the information in question by the reader will render any resulting actions solely under their purview. There are no scenarios in which the publisher or the original author of this work can be in any fashion deemed liable for any hardship or damages that may befall them after undertaking information described herein.! & Additionally, the information in the following pages is intended only for informational purposes and should thus be thought of as universal. As befitting its nature, it is presented without assurance regarding its prolonged validity or interim quality. Trademarks that are mentioned are done without written consent and can in no way be considered an endorsement from the trademark holder.

Table of content:

Breackfast..**13**

    Berry-Coconut Smoothie Bowl............................14

    Cinnamon Walnut Granola................................. 15

    Spinach Artichoke Egg Casserole.........................17

    Coconut and Chia Pudding.................................19

    Spanakopita Frittata..21

    Tropical Yogurt Kiwi Bowl..................................23

    Turkey Sausage Breakfast Muffins.......................24

    Vegetable Breakfast Skillet.................................26

    Parmesan Broiled Flounder................................28

    Grilled Chicken Platter......................................29

    Balsamic Chicken...31

    Healthy Avocado Toast......................................33

    Green Goddess Bowl with Avocado Cumin Dressing...34

    Muffins of Savory Egg.......................................36

    Cottage Cheese Pancakes..................................38

Lunch..**40**

    Berry Apple Cider...41

    Cacciatore Style Chicken...................................43

    Chicken and Sausage Gumbo.............................45

    Thai Peanut, Carrot, and Shrimp Soup.................47

    Mediterranean Spinach Salad.............................49

    Toasted Buckwheat Tabbouleh...........................51

    Rainbow Bean Salad...53

    Crunchy Strawberry Salad.................................55

    Spanish Cauliflower "Rice"................................56

    Chicken-Celery Root Puree..58

    Asparagus Pita Rounds..60

    Rosemary Salmon With Veggies..................................62

    Shrimp Feta And Tomatoes..64

    Amish Coleslaw..66

    Sage Beef..68

Dinner..69

    Wholesome Broccoli Pork Chops................................70

    Crunchy Crusted Salmon..72

    Tomato Steak Kebabs..74

    Beef steaks with green asparagus..............................81

    Lemon Chicken with Basil..83

    Low Carb Rice With Cauliflower................................85

    Salsa Over Chicken..86

    Shrimp-Peach Kabobs..88

    Beef With Barley & Veggies......................................90

    Roasted Tomato Brussels Sprouts.............................92

    Warm Salmon...94

    Crab Cakes...96

    One-Pot Seafood Stew..97

Dessert..100

    Poppy Seed Muffins..100

    Sweet Potato Muffins...103

    Banana Cookies...105

    Pumpkin Bread...107

    Cinnamon Bread...109

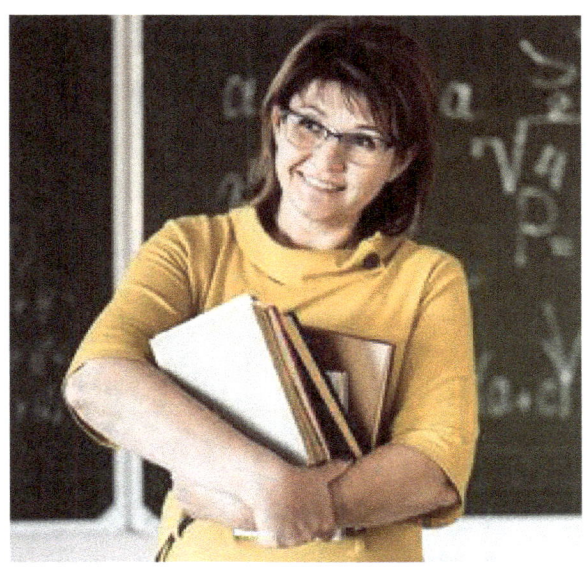

Gena Miller was born in Portland Oregon in 1970 to a wealthy family, Gena has the opportunity to continue her studies away from home, thanks to the economic aid of her father, and for this reason, she decided to attend the renowned university "Columbia University in New York". She had no difficulty in graduating in 1998 with top marks, winning a scholarship in "nutritional sciences" which allowed her to find a job at the university as a lecturer. Gena took her profession very much to heart and saw in teaching the possibility of giving her students the necessary tools to establish a healthy and wholesome lifestyle, drawing up for them real nutritional plans with tasty and healthy recipes. It was her students who encouraged her to start writing "health and wellness" books. The first books were a success and were a stimulus for many people so Gena soon became a successful writer, her experience and love for others led her to understand the real needs of people with food problems and the difficulties they had in approaching food, Gena managed more and more to give the right amount of nutritional value and good taste to her dishes creating delicious and easy recipes appreciated by all.

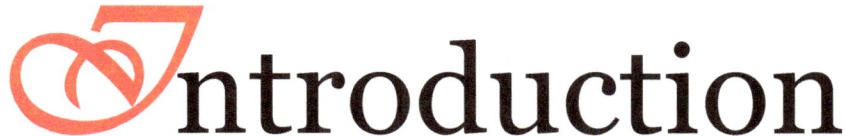
Introduction

Diabetes is a disease in which blood glucose or sugar levels are higher than average. People with diabetes are advised to stay away from certain foods to manage or reverse their condition. But sometimes it's hard to know what to eat and what to avoid so you don't put yourself at risk. This book is tailor-made to present you with several delicious recipes and carefully compiled. In addition to the fantastic meal plan in this book, it is also filled with a detailed and easy procedure to make your own recipes. I'm sure you're looking for a book that explains everything you need to know about your condition and meals to help you manage your condition, is that right? You have chosen the right book. Chapter One WHAT IS DIABETES? Diabetes is a condition in which the pancreas produces insufficient insulin. This means the body is unable to convert food into energy as it should. The body's lack of insulin or its improper use results in high glucose levels that cause abnormal carbohydrate metabolism. Insulin and its activity in the body Insulin is a hormone, and it is produced in the pancreas. It plays a significant role in the control and distribution of energy in the body. It regulates the way the body converts and uses sugar in these simple steps: After food intake (mainly carbohydrates), sugar digests into the bloodstream, which initiates insulin production by the pancreas. The insulin produced circulates throughout the body, helping the sugar enter the cells to provide energy. This leaves less sugar in the bloodstream. The reduction of sugar in the bloodstream causes the pancreas to produce less insulin. Most diabetics have Type II, with one estimate showing that about 90% of diabetes cases are classified as Type II. This is different from the more severe Type 1 diabetes, which requires insulin and is usually treated with medication or by modifying food intake. Some of the risk factors for Type II diabetes are: Older age Obesity History of gestational diabetes Family history of diabetes Impaired glucose tolerance Lack of regular exercise Poor diet In addition to the factors listed above, other factors such as certain races and ethnicities are more likely to develop diabetes. Let's say you are African American, Latino, Native American or Asian American. In this case, you may have a slightly higher chance of developing type II diabetes. There are some cases in pregnancy where the woman develops diabetes. This condition is known as gestational diabetes. It is likely to go away by the end of the pregnancy. However, there is a high chance for a woman who develops gestational diabetes to develop diabetes later in life. This condition occurs more often in blacks, Asians, Hispanics, and American Indians. Finally, there is also a huge chance of having diabetes if your family has it in their history.

Breackfast

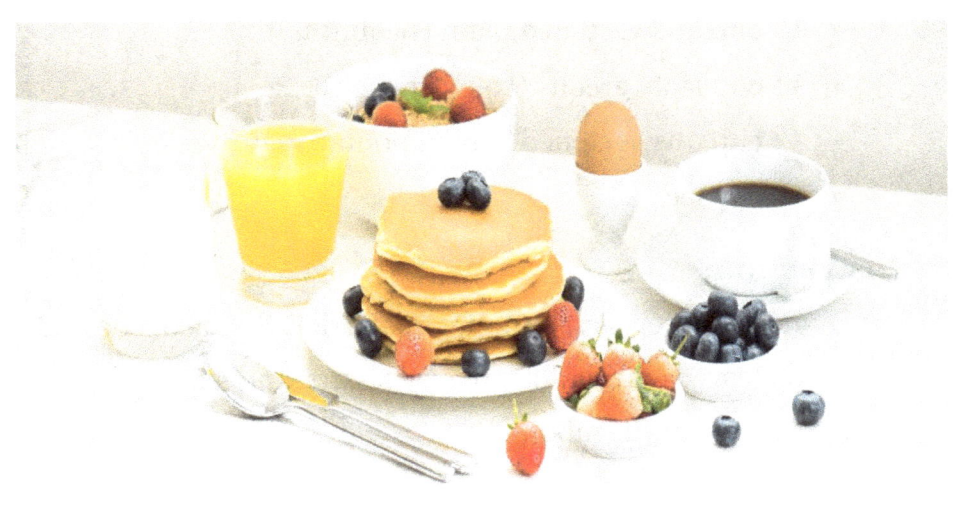

Berry-Coconut Smoothie Bowl

Prep time: 5 minutes
Cook time: 0 minutes
Serves: 2
Ingredients:

- ½ cup mixed berries (blueberries, strawberries, blackberries)
- 1 tablespoon ground flaxseed
- 2 tablespoons unsweetened coconut flakes
- ½ cup unsweetened plain coconut milk
- ½ cup leafy greens (kale, spinach)
- ¼ cup unsweetened vanilla nonfat yogurt
- ½ cup ice

Instruction:
1. In a blender jar, combine the berries, flaxseed, coconut flakes, coconut milk, greens, yogurt, and ice.
2. Process until smooth.
3. Serve.

Nutrition facts:| fat: 15g | protein: 8g | carbs: 8g | sugars: 3g | fiber: 4g | sodium: 24mg

Cinnamon Walnut Granola

Prep time: 10 minutes

Cook time: 30 minutes

Serves 16

Ingredients:
- 4 cups rolled oats
- 1 cup walnut pieces
- ½ cup pepitas
- ¼ teaspoon salt
- 1 teaspoon ground cinnamon
- 1 teaspoon ground ginger
- ½ cup coconut oil, melted
- ½ cup unsweetened applesauce
- 1 teaspoon vanilla extract
- ½ cup dried cherries

Instructions:
1. Preheat the oven to 350°F (180°C).
2. Line a baking sheet with parchment paper.
3. In a large bowl, toss the oats, walnuts, pepitas, salt, cinnamon, and ginger.
4. In a large measuring cup, combine the coconut oil, applesauce, and vanilla.
5. Pour over the dry mixture and mix well.
6. Transfer the mixture to the prepared baking sheet.

7. Cook for 30 minutes, stirring about halfway through.
8. Remove from the oven and let the granola sit undisturbed until completely cool.
9. Break the granola into pieces, and stir in the dried cherries.
10. Transfer to an airtight container, and store at room temperature for up to 2 weeks.

Nutrition facts: calories: 224 | fat: 15g | protein: 5g | carbs: 20g | sugars: 5g | fiber: 3g | sodium: 30mg

Spinach Artichoke Egg Casserole

Prep time: 10 minutes
Cook time: 35 minutes
Serves 8
Ingredients:
- Nonstick cooking spray
- 1 (10-ounce / 283-g) package frozen spinach, thawed and drained
- 1 (14-ounce / 397-g) can artichoke hearts, drained
¼ cup finely chopped red bell pepper
- 2 garlic cloves, minced
- 8 eggs, lightly beaten
- ¼ cup unsweetened plain almond milk
- ½ teaspoon salt
- ½ teaspoon freshly ground black pepper
- ½ cup crumbled goat cheese

Instructions:
1. Preheat the oven to 375°F (190°C).
2. Spray an 8-by-8-inch baking dish with nonstick cooking spray.

3. In a large mixing bowl, combine the spinach, artichoke hearts, bell pepper, garlic, eggs, almond milk, salt, and pepper.
4. Stir well to combine.
5. Transfer the mixture to the baking dish.
6. Sprinkle with the goat cheese.
7. Bake for 35 minutes until the eggs are set.
8. Serve warm.

Nutrition facts: Per Serving calories: 105 | fat: 5g | protein: 9g | carbs: 6g | sugars: 1g | fiber: 2g | sodium: 488mg

Coconut and Chia Pudding

Prep time: 5 minutes

Cook time: 0 minutes

Serves: 2

Ingredients:

- 7 ounces (198 g) light coconut milk
- ¼ cup chia seeds
- 3 to 4 drops liquid stevia
- 1 clementine
- 1 kiwi
- Shredded coconut (unsweetened)

Instructions:

1. Start by taking a mixing bowl and adding in the light coconut milk.
2. Add in the liquid stevia to sweeten the milk.
3. Mix well.
4. Add the chia seeds to the milk and whisk until well-combined.
5. Set aside.
6. Peel the clementine and carefully remove the skin from the wedges.
7. Set aside.
8. Also, peel the kiwi and dice it into small pieces.

9. Take a glass jar and assemble the pudding.
10. For this, place the fruits at the bottom of the jar; then add a dollop of chia pudding.
11. Now spread the fruits and then add another layer of chia pudding.
12. Finish by garnishing with the remaining fruits and shredded coconut.

Nutrition facts: per Serving: calories: 486 | fat: 40.5g | protein: 8.5g | carbs: 30.8g | fiber: 15.6g | sugar: 11.6g | sodium: 24mg

Spanakopita Frittata

Prep time: 10 minutes

Cook time: 15 minutes

Serves: 4

Ingredients:

- 2 tablespoons extra-virgin olive oil
- ½ sweet onion, chopped
- 1 red bell pepper, seeded and chopped
- ½ teaspoon minced garlic
- ¼ teaspoon sea salt
- ½ teaspoon freshly ground black pepper
- 8 egg whites
- 2 cups shredded spinach
- ½ cup crumbled low-sodium feta cheese
- 1 teaspoon chopped fresh parsley, for garnish

Instructions:

1. Preheat the oven to 375°F (190°C).
2. Place a heavy ovenproof skillet over medium-high heat and add the olive oil.
3. Sauté the onion, bell pepper, and garlic until softened, about 5 minutes.
4. Season with salt and pepper.

5. Whisk together the egg whites in a medium bowl, then pour them into the skillet and lightly shake the pan to disburse.
6. Cook the vegetables and eggs for 3 minutes, without stirring.
7. Scatter the spinach over the eggs and sprinkle the feta cheese evenly over the spinach.
8. Put the skillet in the oven and bake, uncovered, until cooked through and firm, about 10 minutes.
9. Loosen the edges of the frittata with a rubber spatula, then invert it onto a plate.
10. Garnish with the chopped parsley and serve.

Nutrition facts: per Serving: calories: 146 fat: 10.1g protein: 10.1g carbs: 3.9g fiber: 1.0g sugar: 2.9g sodium: 292mg

Tropical Yogurt Kiwi Bowl

Prep time: 5 minutes

Cook time: 0 minutes

Serves: 2

Ingredients:

- 1½ cups plain low-fat Greek yogurt
- 2 kiwis, peeled and sliced
- 2 tablespoons shredded unsweetened coconut flakes
- 2 tablespoons halved walnuts
- 1 tablespoon chia seeds
- 2 teaspoons honey, divided (optional)

Instructions:

1. Divide the yogurt between two small bowls.
2. Top each serving of yogurt with half of the kiwi slices, coconut flakes, walnuts, chia seeds, and honey (if using).

Nutrition facts: per Serving: calories: 261 fat: 9.1g protein: 21.1g carbs: 23.1g fiber: 6.1g sugar: 14.1g sodium: 84mg

Turkey Sausage Breakfast Muffins

Prep time: 10 minutes

Cook time: 20 minutes

Serves: 2

Ingredients:

- 2 eggs
- 5 egg whites
- 3 breakfast turkey sausage links, cooked according to package directions
- ¼ cup reduced-fat cheddar cheese, shredded
- ½ cup broccoli florets, fresh, chopped
- ¼ teaspoon fresh ground black pepper
- ¼ cup skim milk

Instructions:

1. Preheat oven to 350° Fahrenheit.
2. Coat 6 muffin cups with some cooking spray.
3. Slice turkey sausage into ½ inch pieces.
4. Set aside.
5. In a mixing bowl, whisk your eggs, egg whites, milk and pepper.
6. Stir in the broccoli florets.

7. Pour your egg mixture evenly into muffin cups about ¾ full.
8. Place sausage into each muffin cup, then sprinkle top with some shredded cheese.
9. Place your muffin tray into the preheated oven and bake for 20 minutes or until the muffins are firm in the center.
10. Remove the muffins from the oven, gently go around each muffin, and remove it from the muffin cup using a knife.
11. Serve and enjoy!

Nutrition facts: (per 1/6 of recipe): Calories: 87 Protein: 9g Fat: 5g Carbs: 2g

Vegetable Breakfast Skillet

Prep time: 12 minutes
Cook time: 15 minutes
Serves: 4
Ingredients:
- 1 cup onions, chopped
- 2 tablespoons olive oil
- 1 pound of frozen potatoes, cubed (4 cups)
- 1 (10-ounce) box frozen asparagus cuts, thawed
- 3 cloves garlic, minced
- ½ lb. Mushrooms, fresh and quartered
- 2 large bell peppers (1 red, 1 yellow), chopped sea salt and black fresh ground pepper to taste

Instructions:
1. Add your oil to a large skillet over medium-high heat.
2. Add your potatoes, along with onions and cook for 10 minutes or until potatoes are lightly browned; stir occasionally.
3. Stir in the mushrooms, bell peppers and garlic, cooking for another 5 minutes or until the peppers are tender, stirring often.

4. Add your asparagus, sea salt and black pepper, cook, until cooked through.
5. Serve and enjoy!

Nutrition facts: (per 1/6 of recipe): Calories: 143 Fat: 5g Protein: 5g Carbs: 22g

Parmesan Broiled Flounder

Prep time: 10 min
Cook time: 6-8 min
Serves: 4
Ingredients:
- 2 (4-oz) flounder
- 1,5 tbsp Parmesan cheese (grated)
- 1,5 tbsp mayonnaise (reduced-fat)
- 1/8 tsp soy sauce
- 1/4 tsp chili sauce
- 1/8 tsp salt-free lemon-pepper seasoning

Instructions:
1. Preheat flounder.
2. Mix cheese, reduced-fat mayonnaise, soy sauce, chili sauce, seasoning.
3. Put fish on a baking sheet coated with cooking spray, sprinkle with salt and pepper.
4. Spread Parmesan mixture over flounder.
5. Broil 6 to 8 minutes or until a crust appears on the fish.
6. A diabetes diet is natural!
7. Enjoy your meal!

Nutrition facts: (100 g) Calories 200 Protein 20 g Fat 17 g Carbs 7 g

Grilled Chicken Platter

Prep Time: 5 minutes

Cook Time: 10 minutes

Serves: 6

Ingredients:

- 3 large chicken breasts, sliced half lengthwise
- 10-ounce spinach, frozen and drained
- 3-ounce mozzarella cheese, part-skim
- 1/2 a cup of roasted red peppers, cut in long strips
- 1 teaspoon of olive oil
- 2 garlic cloves, minced
- Salt and pepper as needed

Instructions:

1. Preheat your oven to 400 degrees Fahrenheit
2. Slice 3 chicken breast lengthwise
3. Take a non-stick pan and grease with cooking spray
4. Bake for 2-3 minutes each side
5. Take another skillet and cook spinach and garlic in oil for 3 minutes
6. Place chicken on an oven pan and top with spinach, roasted peppers, and mozzarella
7. Bake until the cheese melted Enjoy!

Nutrition facts: Calories: 195; Fat: 7g; Net Carbohydrates: 3g; Protein: 30g

Balsamic Chicken

Prep Time: 10 minutes
Cook Time: 25 minutes
Serves: 6
Ingredients:
- 6 chicken breast halves, skinless and boneless
- 1 teaspoon garlic salt
- Ground black pepper
- 2 tablespoons olive oil
- 1 onion, thinly sliced
- 14- and 1/2-ounces tomatoes, diced
- 1/2 cup balsamic vinegar
- 1 teaspoon dried basil
- 1 teaspoon dried oregano
- 1 teaspoon dried rosemary
- 1/2 teaspoon dried thyme

Instructions:
1. Season both sides of your chicken breasts thoroughly with pepper and garlic salt
2. Take a skillet and place it over medium heat
3. Add some oil and cook your seasoned chicken for 3-4 minutes per side until the breasts are nicely browned

4. Add some onion and cook for another 3-4 minutes until the onions are browned
5. Pour the diced-up tomatoes and balsamic vinegar over your chicken and season with some rosemary, basil, thyme, and rosemary
6. Simmer the chicken for about 15 minutes until they are no longer pink
7. Take an instant-read thermometer and check if the internal temperature gives a reading of 165 degrees Fahrenheit

Nutrition facts: Calories: 196; Fat: 7g; Carbohydrates: 7g; Protein: 23g

Healthy Avocado Toast

Prep Time: 5 minutes

Cook Time: 13 minutes

Serves: 4

Ingredients:

- 1 avocado peeled and seeded
- 2 tbsp. chopped cilantro
- Half lime, juiced
- ½ tbsp. red pepper flakes optional
- Salt and pepper to taste
- 2 slices of wholegrain bread or bread of your choice
- 2 eggs fried, scrambled (optional)

Instructions:

1. Toast 2 wholegrain slices in an oven until they are crispy and golden.
2. Mix and crush the avocado, lime, cilantro, and salt and pepper in a shallow bowl to taste.
3. Spread on all the toasted bread slices with half of the combination.
4. Top with fried poached or scrambled egg, if wished.

Nutrition facts: Calories: 501 Fat: 28g Protein: 16g

Green Goddess Bowl with Avocado Cumin Dressing

Prep Time: 10 minutes
Cook Time: 20 minutes
Serves: 4
Ingredients:

- 3 heaping cups finely sliced kale
- 1 small cup diced broccoli florets
- ½ cup zucchini spiralized noodles
- ½ cup soaked Kelp noodles
- 3 cups tomatoes
- 2 tbsp. hemp seeds

Tahini dressing ingredients:

- 1 small cup sesame butter
- 1 cup alkaline water
- 1 cup freshly extracted lemon
- 1 garlic, finely chopped clove
- ¾ tbsp. pure sea salt
- 1 tbsp. olive oil Bell pepper

Avocado Dressing Ingredients:

- 1 big avocado
- 2 freshly extracted lime
- 1 cup alkaline water

- 1 tbsp. olive oil Bell pepper
- 1 tbsp. powdered cumin

Instructions:
1. Simmer veggies—kale and broccoli for about 4 minutes.
2. Combine noodles and add avocado cumin dressing.
3. Toss for a while.
4. Add tomatoes and combine well.
5. Put the cooked kale and broccoli on a plate, add Tahini dressing, add noodles and tomatoes.
6. Add a couple of hemp seeds to the whole dish and enjoy it.

Nutrition facts: Calories: 109 Protein: 25g Fiber: 17g Sugar: 8g

Muffins of Savory Egg

Prep Time: 12 minutes
Cook Time: 33 minutes
Serves: 6
Ingredients:

- 1 ½ cups water
- 2 tbsp. unsalted butter
- 1 (6 oz.) package Stove,
- Top lower-sodium Stuffing Mix for chicken
- 3 oz. bulk pork sausage
- Cooking spray
- 6 eggs, beaten
- ½ cup (1.5 oz.) Monterey Jack cheese, shredded
- ½ cup finely chopped red bell pepper
- ¼ cup sliced green onions

Instructions:

1. Preheat oven to 400°F.
2. In a medium saucepan, put 1 ½ cups water and butter to a boil.
3. Stir in the blend of stuffing.
4. Cover, detach from heat and leave to stand for 5 minutes; use a fork to fluff.

5. Let stand 10 minutes or before cool enough to hold, uncovered.
6. Cook the sausage in a small skillet over medium-high heat until browned while the stuffing is cooling; stir to crumble.
7. Coat the fingers with a mist for frying.
8. Press approximately ¼ cup stuffing into the bottom and sides of each of the 12 deeply coated muffin cups with cooking oil.
9. Pour the egg uniformly into the cups stuffing.
10. Layer cheese, ham, bell pepper, and green onions equally over the egg if desired.
11. Bake for 18 to 20 minutes at 400°F or until the centers are centered.
12. Let it stand before serving for 5 minutes.
13. Run a thin, sharp knife along the edges to loosen the muffin cups.
14. Delete from the casseroles.
15. Immediately serve.

Nutrition facts: Calories: 292 Fat: 16.7g Protein: 14.6g

Cottage Cheese Pancakes

Prep time: 10 minutes
Cook time: 8 minutes
Serves: 2
Ingredients:
- Better Baking Mix, 1 3/4 cups
- Sugar, 1 tablespoon
- Water, 1 cup
- Egg, slightly beaten, 1
- Canola oil, 1-2 tablespoon
- Cottage cheese, 1/2 cup
- Grated lemon peel, 1-2 teaspoons

Instructions:
1. Preheat a frying pan to medium flame.
2. In a big mixing bowl, combine baking powder with some sugar.
3. Now make a well within the middle of the mixture.
4. Add the water, egg, followed by oil, cottage cheese, including lemon peel in the mixing bowl.
5. With a wire brush, combine the mixture until it becomes smooth.
6. Pour batter onto a pan with a 1/4-cup measurement or spoon.

7. Fry pancakes on a pan unless golden brown, rotating once.
8. It's ready.

Nutritional Facts: Fat: 6g, Net Carbs: 37g, Protein: 12g, Sodium: 547mg

Lunch

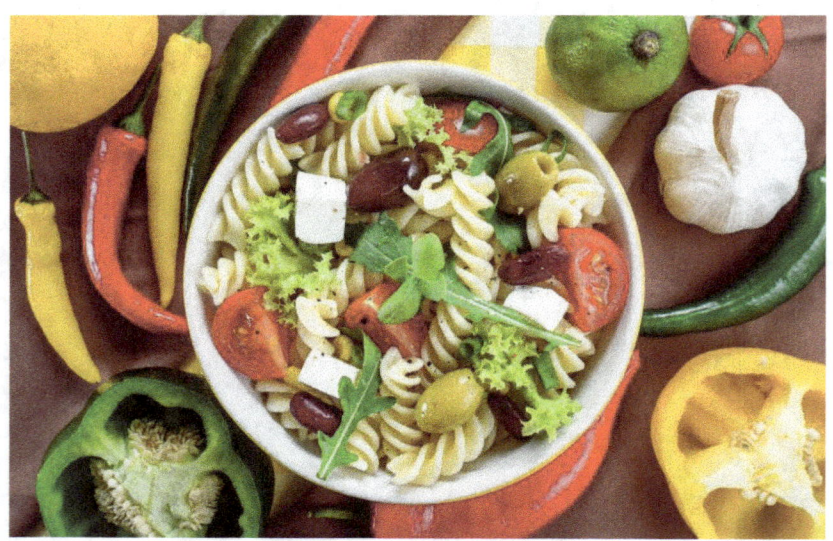

Berry Apple Cider

Prep Time: 15 minutes
Cook Time: 3 hours
Serves: 3
Ingredients:

- 4 cinnamon sticks, cut into 1-inch pieces
- 1½ teaspoons whole cloves
- 4 cups apple cider
- 4 cups low-calorie cranberry-raspberry juice drink
- 1 medium apple

Instructions:

1. To make the spice bag, cut out a 6-inch square from double thick, pure cotton cheesecloth.
2. Put in the cloves and cinnamon, then bring the corners up, tie it closed using a clean kitchen string that is pure cotton.
3. In a 3 1/2- 5-quart slow cooker, combine cranberry-raspberry juice, apple cider, and the spice bag.
4. Cook while covered over low heat setting for around 4-6 hours or on a high heat setting for 2-2 1/2 hours.

5. Throw out the spice bag. Serve right away or keep it warm while covered on warm or low-heat setting up to 2 hours, occasionally stirring.
6. Garnish each serving with apples (thinly sliced).

Nutrition facts: 89 Calories; 22g Carbohydrate; 19g Sug

Cacciatore Style Chicken

Prep Time: 10 minutes
Cook Time: 4 hours
Serves: 6
Ingredients:

- 2 cups sliced fresh mushrooms
- 1 cup sliced celery
- 1 cup chopped carrot
- 2 medium onions, cut into wedges
- 1 green, yellow, or red sweet peppers
- 4 cloves garlic, minced
- 12 chicken drumsticks
- ½ cup chicken broth
- ¼ cup dry white wine
- 2 tablespoons quick-cooking tapioca
- 2 bay leaves
- 1 teaspoon dried oregano, crushed
- 1 teaspoon sugar
- ½ teaspoon salt
- ¼ teaspoon pepper
- 1 (14.5 ounce) can diced tomatoes
- 1/3 cup tomato paste   Hot cooked pasta or rice

Instructions:

1. Mix garlic, sweet pepper, onions, carrot, celery and mushrooms in a 5- or 6-qt. slow cooker.
2. Cover veggies with the chicken.
3. Add pepper, salt, sugar, oregano, bay leaves, tapioca, wine and broth.
4. Cover.
5. Cook for 3–3 1/2 hours on high-heat setting.
6. Take chicken out; keep warm.
7. Discard bay leaves.
8. Turn to high-heat setting if using low-heat setting.
9. Mix tomato paste and undrained tomatoes in.
10. Cover.
11. Cook on high-heat setting for 15 more minutes.
12. Serving: Put veggie mixture on top of pasta and chicken.

Nutrition facts: 324 Calories; 7g Sugar; 35g Carbohydrate

Chicken and Sausage Gumbo

Prep Time: 6 minutes
Cook Time: 4 hours
Serves: 5
Ingredients:

- 1/3 cup all-purpose flour
- 1 (14 ounce) can reduced-sodium chicken broth
- 2 cups chicken breast
- 8 ounces smoked turkey sausage links
- 2 cups sliced fresh okra
- 1 cup water
- 1 cup coarsely chopped onion
- 1 cup sweet pepper
- ½ cup sliced celery
- 4 cloves garlic, minced
- 1 teaspoon dried thyme
- ½ teaspoon ground black pepper
- ¼ teaspoon cayenne pepper
- 3 cups hot cooked brown rice

Instruction:

1. To make the roux: Cook the flour upon a medium heat in a heavy medium-sized saucepan, stirring periodically, for roughly 6 minutes or until the flour browns.
2. Take off the heat and slightly cool, then slowly stir in the broth.
3. Cook the roux until it bubbles and thickens up.
4. Pour the roux in a 3 1/2- or 4-quart slow cooker, then add in cayenne pepper, black pepper, thyme, garlic, celery, sweet pepper, onion, water, okra, sausage, and chicken.
5. Cook the soup covered on a high setting for 3 - 3 1/2 hours.
6. Take the fat off the top and serve atop hot cooked brown rice.

Nutrition facts: 230 Calories; 3g Sugar; 19g Protein

Thai Peanut, Carrot, and Shrimp Soup

Prep Time: 10 minutes
Cook Time: 10 minutes
Serves: 4
Ingredients:

- 1 tablespoon coconut oil
- 1 tablespoon Thai red curry paste
- ½ onion
- 3 garlic cloves
- 2 cups chopped carrots
- ½ cup whole unsalted peanuts
- 4 cups low-sodium vegetable broth
- ½ cup unsweetened plain almond milk
- ½ pound shrimp,
- Minced fresh cilantro, for garnish

Instructions:

1. In a big pan, heat up oil over medium-high heat until shimmering.
2. Cook curry paste, stirring continuously, for 1 minute.

3. Add the onion, garlic, carrots, and peanuts to the pan, and continue to cook for 2 to 3 minutes.
4. Boil broth.
5. Reduce the heat to low and simmer for 5 to 6 minutes.
6. Purée the soup until smooth and return it to the pot.
7. Over low heat, pour almond milk and stir to combine.
8. Cook shrimp in the pot for 2 to 3 minutes.
9. Garnish with cilantro and serve.

Nutrition facts: 237 Calories; 17g Carbohydrates; 6g Sugars

Mediterranean Spinach Salad

Prep time: 15 min
Cook time: 20 minutes
Serves: 4
Ingredients:

- 1 bag baby spinach, washed and dried
- 4-5 spring onions, finely chopped
- 1 cucumber, peeled and cut
- 1/2 cup walnuts, halved and roasted
- 1/3 cup yogurt
- 2 tbsp red wine vinegar
- 3 tbsp extra virgin olive oil salt and black pepper, to taste

Instructions:

1. Whisk yogurt, olive oil and vinegar in a small bowl.
2. Place the baby spinach leaves in a large salad bowl.
3. Add the onions, cucumber and walnuts.
4. Season with black pepper and salt, stir, and toss with the dressing.

Nutrition facts: calories: 136 fat: 11.83g protein: 3.04g carbs: 5.77g fiber: 1.7g sodium: 147mg 124.

Toasted Buckwheat Tabbouleh

Prep time: 10 minutes

Cook time: 20 minutes

Serves: 4

Ingredients

- 1 cup kasha (toasted buckwheat groats)
- 1 tablespoon olive oil
- 2 each onion, peeled and chopped
- 1 clove garlic, minced, or to taste
- 1 cucumber, peeled and diced
- 3/4 cup chopped fresh parsley
- 6 tablespoons chopped fresh mint
- 1 lemon, juiced
- 1 pinch dried mixed herb

Instructions

1. Rinse buckwheat groats.
2. Bring a saucepan of water to a boil, sprinkle in the buckwheat groats, and simmer until buckwheat is tender, about 10 minutes.
3. Drain and cool.

4. Heat olive oil in a skillet over medium heat; cook and stir onions and garlic until onion is translucent, 5 to 8 minutes.
5. Set aside to cool.
6. Lightly toss cucumber, parsley, mint, lemon juice, and mixed herbs in a large salad bowl until thoroughly combined; stir in cooked buckwheat and onion mixture.

Nutrition facts: calories: 575 fat: 29.88g protein: 62.45g carbs: 11.25g fiber: 1.9g sodium: 139mg

Rainbow Bean Salad

Prep Time: 15 minutes
Cook Time: 0 minute
Serves: 5
Ingredients:

- 1 (15 oz.) can low-sodium black beans
- 1 avocado, diced
- 1 cup cherry
- 3 tomatoes, halved
- 1 cup chopped baby spinach
- ½ cup red bell pepper
- ¼ cup jicama
- ½ cup scallions
- ¼ cup fresh cilantro
- 2 tbsp. lime juice
- 1 tbsp. extra-virgin olive oil
- 2 garlic cloves, minced
- 1 tsp. honey
- ¼ tsp. salt
- ¼ tsp. freshly ground black pepper

Instruction:

1. Mix black beans, avocado, tomatoes, spinach, bell pepper, jicama, scallions, and cilantro.
2. Blend lime juice, oil, garlic, honey, salt, and pepper.
3. Add to the salad and toss.
4. Chill for 1 hour before serving.

Nutrition facts: Calories: 169 Carbohydrates: 22g Sugar: 3g

Crunchy Strawberry Salad

Prep Time: 10 minutes

Cook Time: 0 minutes

Serves: 5

Ingredients:

- 0.6 lb. romaine lettuce leaves, roughly torn
- 0.6 lb. strawberries, sliced
- 0.2 lb. nuts of choice

Instructions:

1. In a large mixing bowl add strawberry slices, lettuce, and nuts; toss to combine.
2. Add to a serving bowl.

Nutrition facts: Calories: 94 Fat: 0.3g Protein: 11g

Spanish Cauliflower "Rice"

Prep time: 10 minutes
Cook time: 20 minutes
Serves: 4
Ingredients:

- Large size cauliflower,
- 1 Chicken breasts,
- 1.5 pound Salt,
- 1/2 teaspoon Pepper,
- 1/2 teaspoon Canola oil,
- 1-2 tablespoons Diced green pepper,
- 1 Diced small onion,
- 1 Chopped garlic clove,
- 1 Tomato juice,
- 1-1/2 cup Ground cumin,
- 1-1/4 teaspoon Chopped cilantro,
- 1-1/4 cup Lime juice,
- 1-2 tablespoons

Instructions.

1. Inside a food processor, combine cauliflower in batches unless it matches rice (do not over-mix).
2. Season the chicken with some salt and pepper.
3. Now heat oil inside a large skillet on a medium-high flame; cook chicken breast until lightly browned, approximately 5 minutes.
4. Bake and stir for 3 minutes with the green pepper, diced onion, and garlic.
5. Now bring to a simmer with the tomato juice and ground cumin.
6. Bake over moderate flame for 8-11 minutes, just until cauliflower becomes tender while stirring occasionally.
7. Whisk in the cilantro with lime juice.

Nutrition Facts Fat: 7g, Net Carbs: 15g, Protein: 28g, Sodium: 492mg

Chicken-Celery Root Puree

Prep time: 30 minutes
Cook time: 15 minutes
Serving: 4
Ingredients:

- Debone Chicken breast,
- 4 Pepper,
- 1/2 teaspoon Salt,
- 1/4 teaspoon Canola oil,
- 3-4 teaspoons Chopped celery root,
- 3-4 cups Sliced butternut squash,
- 2-3 cups Diced small onion,
- 1 Chopped garlic cloves,
- 2 Apple juice,
- sugar-free,

Instructions:

1. Season the chicken with some salt and pepper.
2. Inside a big non-stick pan lined with cooking spray, warm 2 teaspoons canola oil over medium flame.
3. Brown all sides of the chicken.
4. Remove the chicken from the plate.

5. Heat the remaining oil in the same pan over moderate heat.
6. Include celery, butternut squash, and diced onion; cook while stirring until the squash is crispy and tender.
7. Bake for 1 minute more after adding the garlic.
8. Return the chicken to the pan and add the apple juice.
9. Now bring to a simmer.
10. Reduce heat to low; boil, covered, for 13-14 minutes, or when a digital thermometer inserted into the chicken reaches 165°Fahrenheit.
11. Remove the chicken and keep warm.
12. Allow the veggies mixture to cool slightly.
13. Inside a food processor, pulse the veggies mixture until smooth.
14. Transfer to the pan and heat properly.
15. Serve with chicken.

Nutritional Facts Fat: 8g, Net Carbs: 28g, Protein: 37g, Sodium: 348mg

Asparagus Pita Rounds

Prep time: 10 minutes
Cook time: 10 minutes
Serving: 3
Ingredients:

- Sliced asparagus, 2 cups
- Olive oil, 2 teaspoons
- Garlic cloves, minced, 2
- Pitas, 4
- Plum tomatoes, 3
- Dried basil, 1 teaspoon
- Salt, 1/4 teaspoon
- Pre-shredded parmesan cheese, 6 tablespoons

Instructions.

1. Preheat the oven to 450°F. Covered, steam asparagus for 2 minutes, or till crisp-tender.
2. Drain after rinsing with cool water.
3. Combine the oil and the garlic cloves.
4. Brush pitas with olive oil.
5. Place tomato slices and the asparagus on pita bread.
6. Season with basil, some pepper, and salt to taste.

7. Evenly sprinkle with the Parmesan cheese.
8. Bake for about 7 to 8 minutes, just until the edges are golden.

Nutritional Facts Fat: 5g, Net Carbs: 40g, Protein: 10g, Sodium: 601mg

Rosemary Salmon With Veggies

Prep time: 10 minutes
Cook time: 20 minutes
Serving: 4
Ingredients:

- Salmon fillets, 1-1/2 pounds
- Olive oil, 2 tablespoons
- Balsamic vinegar, 2 tablespoons
- Fresh rosemary, 2 teaspoons
- Garlic clove, 1
- Salt1/2 teaspoon
- Fresh asparagus, 1 pound
- Sweet red pepper, 1
- Pepper,1/4 teaspoon
- Lemon wedges

Instructions:

1. Heat oven to about 410F.
2. Place the salmon in a 18x12x1-inch baking pan that has been oiled using some cooking oil.

3. Combine the oil, garlic, salt, vinegar, and rosemary in a mixing bowl.
4. Pour half of the sauce over the salmon.
5. In a big mixing cup, combine the asparagus with red pepper and Drizzle with the leftover oil mixture, and combine well.
6. After that, arrange salmon in the pan and season with pepper.
7. Now bake the flakes for about 13 to 17 minutes or till they become soft.
8. Serve immediately with some lemon wedges and enjoy.

Nutritional Facts: Fat: 23g, Net Carbs: 7g, Protein: 31g, Sodium: 388mg

Shrimp Feta And Tomatoes

Prep time: 10 minutes
Cook time: 20 minutes
Serving: 6
Ingredients:

- Olive oil, 3 tablespoons
- Finely chopped shallots, 2
- Crushed red pepper flakes, 1/2 teaspoon
- Sweet paprika, 1/4 teaspoon
- Uncooked large size shrimp, 2 pounds
- Crumbled feta cheese, 2/3 cup
- Minced fresh mint2 teaspoons
- Hot cooked rice, 1 bowl
- Garlic cloves, 2
- Chopped plum tomatoes, 6
- Chicken broth, 1/2 cup
- Dried oregano, 1 tablespoon
- Salt, 1/2 teaspoon

Instructions:

1. Start with Heating some oil in a large size skillet over medium-high flame.

2. Now Cook the shallots with garlic, constantly stirring, until the shallots and garlic are soft.
3. Then bring the tomatoes, chicken broth, oregano, salt, and black pepper to a simmer.
4. Reduce heat to low and cook, uncovered, for 4-5 minutes or until the shrimp turn yellow.
5. After stirring in the shrimp and cheese, finally, cook for 3 minutes more to blend the flavor.
6. Mix in the mint.
7. Serve with potatoes.

Nutritional Facts: Fat: 11g, Net Carbs: 8g, Protein: 28g, Sodium: 480mg

Amish Coleslaw

Prep time: 15 minutes
Cook time: 0 minutes
Serving: 2
Ingredients:

- Torn cabbage, 3.5 cups
- Torn carrots, 3/2 cup
- Chopped celery, 1/2 cup
- Chopped onion, 1/4 cup
- Skimmed mayonnaise, 1/2 cup
- Lemon-pepper seasoning, 1/3 teaspoon
- Horseradish, jarred, 2.5 teaspoons
- Splenda, 2 packets
- White vinegar, 1.5 tablespoons
- Celery seed, 1.5 teaspoons

Instructions:

1. Combine the first 4 ingredients inside a mixing bowl.
2. Combine mayonnaise, followed by lemon-pepper seasoning, then horseradish, Splenda, white vinegar, including celery seed inside a shallow bowl.
3. Now add to the prepared cabbage mixture.

4. Chill, covered, for 60 minutes.
5. Serve right away.

Nutritional Facts Fat: 2g, Net Carbs: 7g, Protein: 1g, Sodium: 198mg

Sage Beef

Preparation Time: 10 minutes
Cooking Time: 30 minutes
Servings: 4
Ingredients:

- 2 lbs. beef stew meat, cubed
- 1 tbsp. sage, chopped
- 2 tbsps. butter, melted
- ½ tsp. coriander, ground
- ½ tbsp. garlic powder
- 1 tsp. Italian seasoning
- Salt and black pepper to the taste

Instructions:

1. In the air fryer's pan, mix the beef with the sage, melted butter, and the other ingredients, introduce the pan in the fryer and cook at 360°F for 30 minutes.
2. Divide everything between plates and serve.

Nutrition Facts: Calories: 290 Fat: 11 g Fiber: 6 g Carbs: 20 g Protein: 29 g

Dinner

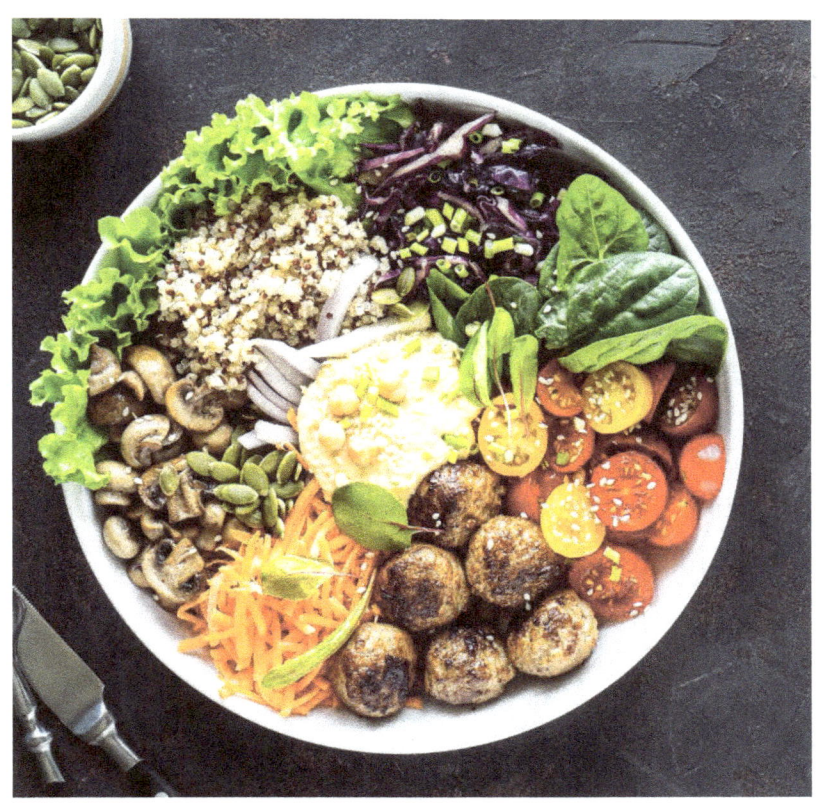

Wholesome Broccoli Pork Chops

Prep Time: 10–15 minutes

Cooking time 10 minutes

Servings: 4

Ingredients

- 1½ tablespoons canola oil (divided)
- ¼ teaspoon red pepper flakes, crushed
- 1 clove garlic, minced
- 1 pound pork loin chops, boneless and divided into
- 4 equal parts 2 cups broccoli florets
- 2 tablespoons + 1 teaspoon reduced-sodium soy sauce
- 2 tablespoons water
- 3 tablespoons rice wine vinegar
- 2 tablespoons cilantro, chopped

Instructions

1. Add the water, soy sauce, vinegar, red pepper, garlic, and 1 tablespoon of the canola oil to a mixing bowl.
2. Mix well. Add the pork chops and combine well. Refrigerate for 20–30 minutes to marinate. Steam the

broccoli florets over boiling water for 5 minutes; drain and set aside.
3. Heat the remaining ½ tablespoon of canola oil over medium heat in a medium saucepan or skillet.
4. Add the pork chops (reserve the marinade) and stir-cook for 4–5 minutes until evenly brown. Transfer the chops to a serving platter.
5. In another saucepan, boil the reserved marinade.
6. Cover and simmer the mixture over low heat for about 2–3 minutes until it thickens.
7. Pour it over the pork chops; top with chopped cilantro and serve with cooked broccoli on the side.

Nutrition facts:: Calories 235, Fat 13 g, Total carbs 5 g, Sugar 1 g, Protein 23 gSodium 480 mg

Crunchy Crusted Salmon

Prep Time: 5–10 minutes

Cook Time: 12–15 minutes

Servings 5

Ingredients

- 2 slices whole-wheat bread, torn into pieces
- 4 teaspoons honey
- 2 teaspoons canola oil
- 3 tablespoons finely chopped walnuts
- 4 (4-ounce) salmon fillets
- 4 teaspoons Dijon mustard
- ½ teaspoon dried thyme

Directions

1. Preheat the oven to 400°F (200°C).
2. Grease a baking sheet with some cooking spray.
3. Place the salmon over the baking sheet.

4. Combine the mustard and honey in a bowl. Brush the salmon with the honey mixture.
5. Add the bread pieces to a blender or food processor and blend to make fine crumbs. Add the crumbs and walnuts to a mixing bowl.
6. Mix well. Add the thyme and canola oil; combine again.
7. Press the mixture over the salmon and bake for 12–15 minutes until the topping is evenly brown and the salmon is easy to flake.
8. Serve warm.

Nutrition facts: Calories 295 Fat 17 g Total carbs 13 g Sugar 7 g, Protein 22 g Sodium 243 mg

Tomato Steak Kebabs

Prep Time: 10–15 minutes

Cook Time 10 minutes

Servings: 4

Ingredients

- 1 teaspoon Dijon mustard
- 1 pound top sirloin steak, cut into 1-inch cubes
- ¼ cup balsamic vinaigrette
- 2 cups cherry tomatoes
- ¼ cup barbecue sauce

Directions

1. Add the barbecue sauce, vinaigrette and mustard to a mixing bowl; mix well.
2. Set aside ¼ of the mixture.
3. Add the beef and coat well.
4. Take four metal or soaked wooden skewers and thread them alternately with tomatoes and beef pieces.
5. Preheat the grill to medium-high heat.

6. Grease the grill rack with cooking spray.
7. Grill the skewers for 6–8 minutes until the beef is tender.
8. When 3–4 minutes remain, begin basting frequently with the reserved mixture.

Nutrition facts: Calories 194, Fat 7 g, Total carbs 7 gSugar 5 g, Protein 25 g, Sodium 288 mg

Green omelette with smoked salmon

Prep Time: 10 minutes

Cook Time: 5 minutes

Servings: 2

Ingredients

- ½ organic cucumber
- Sea salt
- 50 g of salmon, smoked
- 1 box of garden cress
- 20 g of dill
- 3 organic eggs
- pepper, freshly ground
- 2 tbsp. mineral water
- 80 grams of kefir
- 2 tbsp. olive oil for frying

Direction:

1. Wash the cucumber thoroughly and cut into thin slices. Set aside a few slices. Spread the rest on two plates and sprinkle with sea salt and pepper.

2. Cut the smoked salmon into bite-sized pieces.
3. Cut off the cress, wash, dry and finely chop the dill.
4. Put the eggs together with the sea salt, pepper, mineral water and kefir in a tall container and stir well with a whisk.
5. Then mix in the dill. Heat two small pans with oil.
6. Put half of the egg mixture into each pan and let it set over a low heat for about 3–4 minutes.
7. Top the finished omelets with the salmon, cucumber slices (the ones that were set aside) and cress.
8. Finally, fold up the omelettes, cut in half and arrange on the plates with the cucumber slices.
9. Note: Cucumbers have hardly any calories, are rich in important nutrients and are 96 % water. This means that they can also be eaten in large quantities.

Nutrition facts: Calories: 382 kcal Protein: 20.57 g Fat: 30.4 g Carbohydrates: 6.04 g

Stuffed tomatoes with quinoa

Prep Time: 10 minutes

Cook Time: 20 minutes

Servings: 2

Ingredients

- 50 g of colorful quinoa
- 2 organic beefsteak tomatoes, large
- 50 g spinach, fresh or frozen
- 1 spring onion
- 50 g paprika, grilled out of the glass
- Walnut oil, as needed
- 1 tsp. white wine vinegar
- Sea salt and black pepper from the mill
- 1 whole grain baguette
- 2 cloves of garlic

Directions

1. Cook the quinoa according to the instructions on the packet, place in a colander and drain. Wash tomatoes, cut off a lid, remove the pulp with a spoon and chop.
2. Sort the spinach and wash it thoroughly.
3. Clean, wash and cut the spring onions into rings.
4. Drain the peppers and cut into small pieces.
5. Heat the oil in a pan, sauté the onions, add the spinach and let it collapse over a low heat.
6. Add paprika and quinoa and cook for another 3 minutes. Season to taste with vinegar, sea salt and pepper.
7. Season the tomatoes from the inside with salt and pepper, add the filling, and put the lid on the tomato.
8. Grease a baking dish a little and put the tomatoes in it, put the oven on the grill and cook for about 15–20 minutes.
9. In the meantime, peel off the garlic, cut the whole wheat baguette into slices, rub with garlic and either roast in a pan with a little oil, toast or also roast in the grill.
10. Serve the filled tomatoes with the wholemeal baguette and enjoy.
11. Note: Quinoa is available in many supermarkets or in health food stores. TIP: If you don't have colorful quinoa, use white.

Nutrition facts: Calories: 202 kcal Protein: 9.85 g Fat: 5.12 g Carbohydrates: 37.67 g

Beef steaks with green asparagus

Prep Time: 15 minutes

Cook Time: 20 minutes

Servings: 4

Ingredients

- 500 g asparagus, green
- 40 g herb butter
- 2 beef fillet steaks (approx. 150 g each)
- 1 dried tomato pickled in oil
- 50 g ricotta
- Sea salt and black pepper
- Herbs, fresh e.g. B. oregano, basil
- 1 tbsp. oil for frying & capers, as desired (optional)

Directions

1. Wash the asparagus and peel the lower ends.
2. Prepare two pieces of baking paper or aluminum foil and spread the asparagus on top.
3. Put the herb butter on the asparagus, close the foil tightly, put on the grill for about 10 - 15 minutes.

4. Dab steaks with a little paper towel, cut a pocket. Drain the tomatoes and cut into small pieces.
5. Put the ricotta and capers in a bowl, wash, dry and chop the herbs and add them as well.
6. Mix everything well and season with sea salt and pepper. Pour the finished cream into the steaks and seal the openings with a toothpick.
7. Finally, season the steaks with sea salt and pepper, brush with the oil and grill depending on the degree of cooking required (approx. 5–8 minutes on each side).
8. Arrange the steaks with the asparagus, add the rest of the cream and serve hot.
9. Note: If you don't have a grill, you can prepare both the asparagus and the steaks in the oven.
10. First fry the steaks briefly in the pan and then finish cooking in the oven.

Nutrition facts: Calories: 339 kcal Protein: 18.91 g Fat: 27.06 g Carbohydrates: 6.31 g

Lemon Chicken with Basil

Prep Time: 10 minutes

Cook Time:1 hour

Servings: 4

Ingredients

- 1 kg chopped chicken
- 2 lemons
- 2 cups basil
- Salt and ground pepper
- 1 tbsp.
- extra virgin olive oil

Direction

1. Put the chicken in a bowl with a jet of extra virgin olive oil.
2. Put salt, pepper, and basil.
3. Bind well and let stand for at least 30 minutes, stirring occasionally.
4. Put the pieces of chicken in the air fryer basket and take the air fryer.
5. Select 30 minutes.
6. Move occasionally.

7. Take out and put another batch.
8. Repeat the same process.

Nutrition facts: Calories: 1,440 Fat: 74.9 g Carbs: 122.0 g Protein: 68.6 g

Low Carb Rice With Cauliflower

Prep time: 3 minutes

Cook time: 7 minutes

Serving: 4

Ingredients

- Medium size Cauliflower
- 1 Coriander
- chopped
- 1 handful

Instructions

1. Remove cauliflower's hard-core stalks and pulse inside a food processor to make rice-sized grains.
2. Place in a bowl, cover with the cling film, and then microwave for 7 minutes on high.
3. Add the coriander and mix well.
4. To make the rice spicier, toss in some toasted cumin seeds.
5. Serve and enjoy!

Nutritional Facts Fat: 1g, Net Carbs: 4g, Protein: 5g, Sodium: 136m

Salsa Over Chicken

Prep time: 10 minutes

Cook time: 15 minutes

Serves: 4

Ingredients

- Fresh peaches
- 1-1/2 cups Chopped cucumber
- 3/4 cup Peach preserves
- 4 tablespoons Red onion
- 3 tablespoons Minced mint
- 1 teaspoon Salt, divided
- 3/4 teaspoon Chicken breast
- 4 Pepper, 1/4 teaspoon

Instructions

1. To make the salsa, add peaches, 3/4 cup of cucumber, 2 teaspoons of preserves, onion, 1 teaspoon mint, and 1/4 teaspoon of salt in a cup.
2. Season the chicken with some pepper and the remaining salt.
3. Grill the chicken for 5 mins, covered, on the finely oiled rack over the medium heat.

4. Grill for 7-9 minutes further, or till a hermometer reads 165° and brush tops with the remaining preserves periodically.
5. Serve with salsa.

Nutritional Facts Fat: 4g, Net Carbs: 20g, Protein: 35g, Sodium: 525mg

Shrimp-Peach Kabobs

Prep time: 10 minutes

Cook time: 10 minutes

Serves: 4

Ingredients

- Brown sugar
- 1 tablespoon Paprika
- 1 teaspoon Ancho chili pepper
- 1 teaspoon Ground cumin
- 1/2 teaspoon Salt
- 1/4 teaspoon Pepper
- 1/4 teaspoon Cayenne pepper
- 1/4 teaspoon Shrimp
- 1 pound Medium peaches
- 3 Green onions, 8
- Cooking spray
- 2 tablespoons Lime wedges

Instructions

1. Mix some brown sugar and the seasonings.
2. Toss the shrimps, peaches, and green onions in a mixing bowl with the brown sugar mixture.

3. Now thread shrimps, peaches, and the green onions on four metal skewers.
4. Spray all sides of the kabobs lightly with the cooking spray for 3-4 mins on either side, covered, over medium heat, or before shrimps turn pink.
5. Squeeze lime wedges on top of the kabobs.
6. Serve and enjoy.

Nutritional Facts Fat: 2g, Net Carbs: 18g, Protein: 20g, Sodium: 289mg

Beef With Barley & Veggies

Prep time: 10 minutes

Cook time: 30 minutes

Serves: 2

Ingredients

- ¾ cup filtered water
- ¼ cup pearl barley
- 2 teaspoons olive oil
- 7 ounces lean ground beef
- 1 cup fresh mushrooms, sliced
- ¾ cup onion, chopped
- 2 cups frozen green beans
- ¼ cup low-sodium beef broth
- 2 tablespoon fresh parsley, chopped

Instructions

1. In a pan, add water, barley and pinch of salt and bring to a boil over medium heat.
2. Now, reduce the heat to low and simmer, covered for about 30-40 minutes or until all the liquid is absorbed.

3. Remove from heat and set aside. In a skillet, heat oil over medium-high heat and cook beef for about 8-10 minutes.
4. Add the mushroom and onion and cook f or about 6-7 minutes.
5. Add the green beans and cook for about 2-3 minutes.
6. Stir in cooked barley and broth and cook for about 3-5 minutes more. Stir in the parsley and serve hot.
7. Meal Prep Tip: Transfer the beef mixture into a large bowl and set aside to cool. Divide the mixture into 2 containers evenly.
8. Cover the containers and refrigerate for 1-2 days.
9. Reheat in the microwave before serving.

Nutritional Facts: Calories 374 Total Fat 11.4 g Saturated Fat 3.1 g Cholesterol 89 mg Total Carbs 32.7g Sugar 1.1 g Fiber 4.2 g Sodium 136 mg Potassium 895 mg Protein 36.6 g

Roasted Tomato Brussels Sprouts

Prep Time: 15 minutes

Cook Time: 20 minutes

Serves: 4

Ingredients

- 1-pound (454 g) Brussels sprouts
- 1 tablespoon extra-virgin olive oil
- ½ cup sun-dried tomatoes
- 2 tablespoons lemon juice
- 1 teaspoon lemon zest

Instructions

1. Set oven 205°C. Prep large baking sheet with aluminum foil.
2. Toss the Brussels sprouts in the olive oil in a large bowl until well coated.
3. Sprinkle with salt and pepper.

4. Spread out the seasoned Brussels sprouts on the prepared baking sheet in a single layer.
5. Roast for 20 minutes, shake halfway through.
6. Remove from the oven then situate in a bowl. Whisk tomatoes, lemon juice, and lemon zest, to incorporate.
7. Serve immediately.

Nutritional Facts: 111 calories 13.7g carbohydrates 4.9g fiber

Warm Salmon

Prep time: 20 min

Cook time: 15 min

Serving: 4

Ingredients

- 400g baby new potato , halved
- 2 salmon fillets , skin on, (about 140g/5oz each)
- small handful black olive (we like Kalamata)
- small handful sundried tomato , chopped
- 1 garlic clove ,
- crushed juice ½ lemon
- 1 tbsp olive oil
- 200g green beans

Instructions:

1. Bring half of a large steamer to a boil, pour in the potatoes, then the salmon fillets, skin side down.
2. Cover and cook for 6-8 minutes until the salmon is cooked through, then set aside.
3. Cook the potatoes for another 5-8 minutes until tender, adding the beans for the last couple of minutes.
4. Drain the vegetables, pour into a bowl.

5. Also add the olives and tomatoes, flake the cooked salmon into pieces, discarding the skin.
6. Whisk the garlic, lemon and oil with some of the dressing, and dissolve with a few drops of water.
7. Pour over the dressing, mix well and serve.

Nutrition facts: 196 calories , 144 milligrams sodium, 0 grams trans fat, 11 grams protein, 2g fat

Crab Cakes

Prep time: 10 minutes
Cook time: 15minutes
Servings: 6
Ingredients:

- 1 egg
- ⅓ cup of finely chopped green or red pepper
- ¼ cup reduced fat mayonnaise
- ⅓ cup low sodium crackers
- 1 tablespoon dry mustard
- 1 teaspoon crushed red pepper or black pepper
- 2 tablespoons lemon juice
- 2 tablespoon vegetable oil
- 1 teaspoon garlic powder

Instructions:

1. Mix up all ingredients.
2. Share into 6 balls and craft out patties.
3. Warm up vegetable oil in pan at average heat (or oven at 350°f).
4. Fry already formed patties 4-5 minutes or bake 15 minutes in oven.
5. Serve while still warm

Nutrition facts: 101 calories, 67 milligrams sodium, 0 grams trans fat, 2 grams protein, 41 milligrams, cholesterol 9 grams total fat

One-Pot Seafood Stew

Prep Time: 5 Minutes

Cook Time: 20 Minutes

Serves: 3

Ingredients

- 2 Garlic Cloves, Pressed
- ½ Pound Shrimp
- 1 Tsp Italian Seasonings
- 1 Celery Stalk, Chopped
- 1 Cup Hot Water
- 2 Tomatoes, Pureed
- 2 Tbsps Dry White Wine
- ½ Tsp Lemon Zest
- ½ Pound Mussels
- 1 Tsp Saffron Threads
- Salt And Ground Black Pepper, To Taste
- ½ Stick Butter, At Room Temperature
- 2 Cups Shellfish Stock
- 2 Onions, Chopped

Instructions:

1. Dissolve The Butter In A Stockpot Over A Normal Heat.
2. Heat The Onion And Garlic Until Aromatic.
3. After That, Stir In Pureed Tomatoes;

4. Cook For About 8 Minutes Or Until Heated Through.
5. Include The Remaining Ingredients And Bring To A Rapid Boil.
6. Decrease The Heat To A Simmer And Heat An Additional 4 Minutes.
7. Ladle Into Individual Bowls And Enjoy Warm.

Nutrition facts : Calories209, Protein 15.2g, Fat 12.6g, Carbs 6.6g, Sugar 3.1g

Dessert

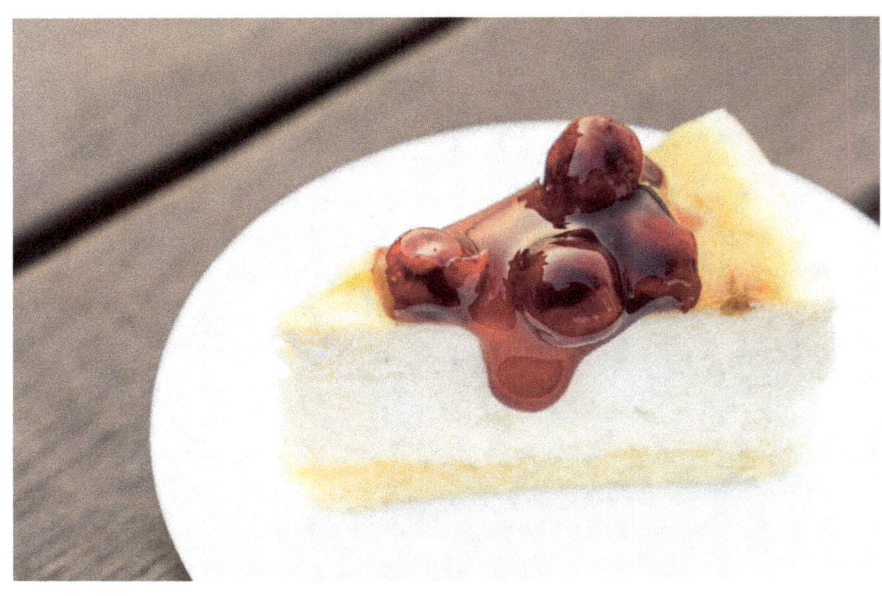

Poppy Seed Muffins

Preparation Time: 7 Minutes
Cooking Time: 32 Minutes
Servings: 6
Ingredients:

- 1 cup almond flour
- 1/2 cup golden flax meal
- 1 teaspoon baking powder
- 1/8 teaspoon salt
- 1 teaspoon poppy seeds
- 1 cup granular Splenda
- 2 tablespoons butter
- 1 teaspoon pure lemon extract
- 1 teaspoon vanilla
- 2 tablespoons heavy cream
- 2 tablespoons water
- 2 eggs

Instructions:

1. Preheat the oven to 350°F.
2. Line 6 muffin cups with liners.
- In a small bowl, stir together the almond flour, flax meal, baking powder, salt, poppy seeds, and granular Splenda, if using.

- In a medium microwave-safe bowl, melt the butter in the microwave.
- Stir in the Splenda, lemon extract, cream, and water.
- Add the dry ingredients and the eggs to the butter mixture.
- Stir with a wooden spoon until well blended.
- Fill muffin cups evenly with the batter.
- Bake 15-20 minutes until the tops are golden brown.
- Let cool for 5 minutes on a rack before removing it from the pan.
- Serve and enjoy!

Nutrition facts: Calories: 128 Total Carbs: 14g Fat: 5g Protein: 12g 76.   No Sugar

Sweet Potato Muffins

Preparation Time: 11 Minutes
Cooking Time: 30 Minutes
Servings: 6
Ingredients:

- 3/4 cup almond meal
- 1 teaspoon baking soda
- 1/4 teaspoon salt
- 1 teaspoon ground cinnamon
- 1/2 teaspoon ground cardamom
- 1/4 teaspoon ground cloves
- 1/4 teaspoon anise powder
- 2/3 cup coconut cream
- 3 tablespoons almond butter
- 4 large eggs, at room temperature
- Zest of 1 orange
- 2 tablespoons vanilla extract
- 1 tablespoon apple cider vinegar
- 1 cup raw grated sweet potato
- 1/2 cup sugar substitute

Instructions:

1. Preheat the oven to 350°F.

2. Line a muffin tin with muffin liners.

3. In a medium bowl, mix almond meal, baking soda, salt, and spices.

4. Mix well.

5. Add the coconut butter and almond butter and mix well again.

6. Add the eggs, zest, vanilla, vinegar, sweet potato, and sweetener.

7. Mix until smooth.

8. Sweeten to taste.

9. Fill muffin cups about 3/4 full with batter.

10. Bake 22-28 minutes, or until a wooden toothpick comes out clean.

Nutrition facts: Calories: 117 Total Carbs: 12g Fat: 3g Protein: 11g 80.

Banana Cookies

Preparation Time: 9 Minutes
Cooking Time: 30 Minutes
Servings: 12
Ingredients:

- 2 1/4 cups flour
- 1 teaspoon baking soda
- 1 teaspoon salt
- 3/4 cup unsweetened applesauce
- 2 egg whites
- 1/2 cup Splenda sugar substitute
- 1/4 cup sugar
- 1/2 cup Splenda brown sugar blend
- 1 medium banana, mashed
- 1 teaspoon vanilla
- 1 1/4 cups semi-sweet chocolate chips
- 4 Marshmallows, shredded

Instructions:

1. Preheat the oven to 350°F.
2. Stir flour, salt, and baking soda in a bowl, then set aside.

3. Beat applesauce, egg whites, and sugars with a mixer.
4. Mix in bananas and vanilla.
5. Slowly add flour mixture to the mixer.
6. Add chocolate chips and marshmallows.
7. Drop by spoonfuls on the cookie sheet.
8. Bake for 15 minutes.

Nutrition facts: Calories: 83 Fat: 2g Carbohydrates: 16g Protein: 1g

Pumpkin Bread

Preparation time: 15 minutes
Cooking time: 65 minutes
Servings 5
Ingredients:

- ¾ Cup of almond flour 2 to 3 egg whites
- 4 Tbsps of pumpkin puree
- 4 Tbsps of almond milk
- 2 Tbsps of Psyllium Husk powder
- 1Teaspoon of baking powder
- 1 Teaspoon of pumpkin spice
- ¼ Teaspoon of salt

Instructions:

1. Preheat your oven to 345 F and then line a medium sized loaf pan with parchment paper.
2. Put a medium pan into the rack of your oven and pour water in that pan.
3. Combine your dry ingredients all together in a deep bowl and mix very well until it is perfectly incorporated.
4. Add the egg whites and the pumpkin puree to your dry mixture.

5.   Pour the almond milk into the mixture and knead it until you form solid dough.

6.   Knead the dough until it becomes dough smooth to the touch and place your dough into the loaf pan you have prepared.

7.   Bake the pumpkin loaf in the Bain-marie for around 60 to 65 minutes.

8.   When a toothpick you insert comes out clean, turn off the heat and remove your loaf pan from the oven.

9.   Let the loaf bread rest for 15 minutes.

10.   Slice and serve.

11.   Enjoy your bread!

Nutrition facts: Calories: 75 | Fat: 4 g | Carbohydrates 2.5g | Fiber: 0.7 g |Protein: 3 g

Cinnamon Bread

Preparation time: 10 minutes
Cooking time: 45 minutes:
Servings: 6
Ingredients:
- 1 and ½ cups of almond flour
- ¾ Teaspoon of baking soda
- ½ Teaspoon of baking powder
- ¼ Teaspoon of salt
- 1 Teaspoon of cinnamon
- ½ Teaspoon of ground all spice
- 4Tbsp of butter
- 2 Large organic eggs
- 1 Cup of avocado puree
- ½ Cup of heavy cream
- ½ Tbsp of grated lemon zest

Instructions:

1. Preheat your oven to 340 F and line a loaf pan with parchment paper; then set it aside.

2. In a deep bowl, combine all together the baking powder, the salt, the lemon zest, the all spice and the cinnamon and mix very well.
3. Pour the butter in a bowl and with a hand mixer beat it until it becomes soft and very smooth.
4. Add in the eggs and the avocado puree then carry on mixing the ingredients.
5. Add your dry mixture and the heavy cream into your batter and mix it very well until it is very well combined.
6. Transfer your batter to your already prepared loaf pan then bake it for around 45 minutes.
7. After around 45 minutes, poke the bread with the knife.
8. Remove your bread from the oven and set it aside to cool on a rack.
9. Set the bread aside to cool down and after that, slice it.
10. Serve and enjoy it!

Nutrition facts: Calories: 173 | Fat: 15 g | Carbohydrates: 2g | Fiber: 2 g | Protein: 6 g

www.ingramcontent.com/pod-product-compliance
Lightning Source LLC
Chambersburg PA
CBHW070931080526
44589CB00013B/1478